Dr. Earl Mindell's

What You Should Know About the Super Antioxidant Miracle

Other Keats titles by Dr. Earl Mindell

Dr. Earl Mindell's Garlic: The Miracle Nutrient
Dr. Earl Mindell's Live Longer and Feel Better
With Vitamins & Minerals

Dr. Earl Mindell's

What You Should Know About the Super Antioxidant Miracle

Earl L. Mindell, R.Ph.

with Virginia L. Hopkins

Keats Publishing, Inc. New Canaan, Connecticut

Dr. Earl Mindell's What You Should Know About the Super Antioxidant Miracle is intended solely for informational and educational purposes, and not as medical advice. Please consult a medical or health professional if you have questions about your health.

Contents

CHAPTER 1

Nature's Neutralizers:
The Antioxidants

Vitamins and minerals are nutrients that are essential to life and to good health, and yet less than 10 percent of Americans meet even the RDA (Recommended Dietary Allowance) of vitamin intake. This leaves more than 90 percent of the population short of essential nutrients. In fact, even the RDA is far short of what you need to stay healthy, indicating only the amount of a nutrient you need to keep from getting diseased. The amounts of nutrients you need for vibrant good health and energy are much higher than the RDA.

Taking antioxidants supplements not only optimizes your health and energy levels, it is a form of health insurance. These miraculous substances also give us a way to protect our bodies from air pollution, pesticides, additives in our food, and radiation, not to mention the effects of aging, stress and illness.

You've probably heard a lot about the best-known antioxidants, vitamins C and E and beta-carotene, but there are other less well-known antioxidants with actions that are even more potent, that I call *super antioxidants*. These substances, while not called vitamins because they aren't essential to life, are powerful weapons in your arsenal of nutritional healing supplements.

Although some, like grapeseed extract, seem to be beneficial for virtually all parts of the body, others, like ginkgo biloba, specifically enhance memory.

1

There are literally hundreds of good scientific studies showing that these super antioxidants can do everything from preventing heart disease and cancer to improving vision and enhancing brain function.

THE MIRACLE OF ANTIOXIDANT POWER

What are these new miracle supplements? Actually, they aren't new, we just know more than we used to about them and how they work in helping to protect our bodies. Let's begin by finding out what's behind antioxidant power. There are hundreds and probably even thousands of antioxidants, most of them found naturally in plants, particularly fresh fruits and vegetables, but also in herbs. Antioxidants are also present to some degree in seafood and in some animal foods. Other antioxidants, such as coenzyme Q10 and glutathione, the body can manufacture itself.

OXIDATION AND FREE RADICALS

What antioxidants do in the body is help neutralize the damage of oxidation. We can think of oxidation as similar to what happens to metal when it rusts, or to an apple when it turns brown. Have you ever prevented a cut-up apple from turning brown by squeezing some lemon juice on it? The vitamin C in the lemon juice is an antioxidant that is stopping the oxidation process. When meat spoils, or oil goes rancid, oxidation is in process.

The word *oxidation* comes from oxygen, an element which is essential to life, but that can be harmful in some forms inside the body. A "good" oxygen molecule has its electrons paired up, making them stable. An unstable or "bad" oxygen molecule has a missing electron, creating what is called a free radical. These unstable oxygen molecules go to war in the body, grabbing onto other cells in their attempt to find another electron and stabilize. This electron can be captured from DNA, cell wall membranes, lipids, proteins, or almost any other tissue component. Every time a free radical stabilizes itself by attacking another cell, it leaves the cell it attacked damaged. That cell becomes unstable and in turn goes after another, creating a chain reaction. This is the process known as oxidation.

The damage free radicals do includes cell mutation that can lead to cancer. Other kinds of damage can contribute to cardiovascular disease, cataracts, macular degeneration, arthritis, diseases affecting the brain, the kidneys, the lungs, the digestive system and the immune system. Free radicals are involved in the damage done by alcoholism, aging, radiation injury, iron overload, and diseases that affect the blood such as strokes. Once the process of oxidation begins, it can be hard to stop, so your best health plan is to prevent it in the first place.

What creates free radicals? First, our bodies naturally produce free radicals as part of our complex interaction with oxygen. Our bodies convert much of the food we eat to sugars. Tiny cellular power plants called mitochondria, which are present in every cell, use these sugars plus oxygen to produce energy. Byproducts of this energy production are free radicals, which if not neutralized by antioxidants, create cellular damage.

Free radicals also play a positive role in the body. They act as chemical messengers, helping in the production of hormones, and activating enzymes which are necessary to nearly every system in the body. Free radicals are used by the immune system to fight off invading bacteria and viruses. They have become a problem largely because of the polluted environment we live in, and our poor diets.

It is excessive free radicals, not balanced properly with antioxidants, that do damage. The ideal body, with ideal nutrition, in an ideal environment, would have the ability to counteract the free radicals it produces with the antioxidants it takes in and produces, and keep them under control. Heavy exercise produces free radicals, but it also has beneficial effects on the body that help counteract them.

PUT ON YOUR ANTIOXIDANT ARMOR AGAINST POLLUTION

There are dozens of environmental causes of free radical production. The biggest culprits we know of are pollutants such as smog, toxins such as chlorine, herbicides and pesticides, radiation, some food additives, cigarette smoke, many prescription drugs, and rancid oil. Furthermore, most Americans eat relatively few fresh fruits and vegetables, one of our main natural sources of antioxidants.

What we have in today's world is a situation where we end up with more free radicals than our bodies can handle. These excess free radicals cause oxidation damage in our bodies. This is where supplements come in.

One of the facts of life in the 1990s is that nearly all of us are exposed to pollutants and toxins every day. From the moment we get up in the morning and shower with chlorinated water (I hope you aren't drinking it!), eat pesticide- and additive-laden food, drive to work breathing in car exhaust and toxic fumes from the interior of our cars, work in a building that's most likely toxic from the chemicals put in paneling and carpets, use machines that emit fumes and radiation, and then return home, where we use pesticides, herbicides, spray cans, and cleaning products with toxic fumes—whew! Enough already! But don't despair—there are ways to fight back.

NATURE'S FREE RADICAL NEUTRALIZERS

The very best way to get your antioxidants and other vitamins is to eat plenty of whole, preferably organic foods. Fresh fruits and vegetables are your primary dietary source of antioxidants. Those highest in antioxidant power are:

- Fresh or frozen broccoli, cauliflower and cabbage. Please don't boil your vegetables and lose most of the nutrients in the water. Steam them or eat them raw! If you don't have one, buy a steamer for a few dollars that fits in most pots. You'll find them in your supermarket or kitchen supply store.
- Dark, leafy green vegetables such as spinach and kale.
- Onions and garlic.
- The "yellow" vegetables such as carrots, sweet potatoes and pumpkins.
- Fresh, whole fruit versus canned or juices.

EAT SOME SEAFOOD FOR OMEGA-3 FATTY ACIDS

Seafood is very high in the omega-3 fatty acids, which can actually *reduce* the damage caused by oxidation. However, since much of our fish is contaminated with pollutants, follow these safe fish-eating rules:

- Rotate the kinds of fish you eat, and don't eat any one kind of fish more than once a week.
- Don't eat fish caught close to shore or in rivers and lakes, which are more likely to be polluted.
- Avoid the skin, which has a higher concentration of toxins.

Although all seafood contains omega-3 fatty acids, the highest concentrations are found in mackerel, salmon, tuna (packed in water, please), herring and sardines. One of my favorite fish is sea bass. Although it's not quite as high in omega-3 fatty acids as the other fish I've listed, it is caught in deep off-shore waters so it's relatively pollutant-free.

Other foods high in omega-3 fatty acids are avocados and almonds.

STEER CLEAR OF RANCID OILS

One of the biggest sources of free radicals in the Western diet is rancid oil. Unfortunately, the processed vegetable oils (corn, safflower, sunflower, soy, etc.) so heavily promoted for good health for the past thirty years have probably been major contributors to disease in this country. They are high in omega-6 fatty acids, which are very unstable and go rancid almost instantly when they are processed. These rancid fats wreak havoc in the body, setting loose a chain reaction of oxidation. Meat also contains omega-6 fatty acids, but if you eat it in moderation, the benefits of the nutrients you receive from it will outweigh the damage of the omega-6.

Please avoid corn, safflower, sunflower, cottonseed and other vegetable oils that are "hydrogenated," "polyunsaturated," or otherwise processed. The hydrogenated oils are synthetic, not-found-in-nature pseudo-saturated oils which are worse for you than the real thing. Even "cold-pressed" vegetable oils are suspect because they go rancid so quickly (most within hours after you open the container). To prevent rancidity, add the contents of a 400 IU vitamin E oil capsule to the bottle of vegetable oil when you open it. Some brands already have vitamin E added.

Olive oil is the only vegetable oil that is low in omega-6 fatty acids and doesn't go rancid quickly. Canola oil is better than most at 60 percent omega-3 fatty acids, but still goes rancid fairly quickly. Look for canola oil with vitamin E added, or add it yourself as I mentioned above.

Coconut oil is a good oil because it is high in stearic acid, which has a neutral effect on cholesterol, doesn't go rancid quickly, and is excellent for baking. I would much rather have you use coconut oil than hydrogenated oils such as Crisco and margarine. I know this flies in the face of mainstream dietary advice, but tropical oils were drummed out of the American diet for political reasons within the food manufacturing industry, not for sound nutritional reasons.

MINIMIZE POLLUTANTS TO KEEP ANTIOXIDANTS AT BAY

- Drink clean water (filtered), 8-10 glasses daily.
- Wash, peel or even scrub fruits and vegetables well and eat organic produce whenever possible.
- As much as possible, eat whole, unprocessed foods without additives and preservatives.
- Read food labels.
- Stand up for your right to work in a pollution-free environment. If you think something at work

is making you sick, pursue it. It could be mold or fungus in the heating or cooling system, fumes from wall paneling or carpets, or a co-worker's cigarette smoke.

- Minimize your use of spray cans, herbicides and pesticides.
- Avoid processed vegetable oils, eat meat in moderation, eat more seafood and more olive oil.

ANTIOXIDANTS AND AGING

Scientists who study aging are increasingly focusing on the cumulative damage done to cellular DNA over time by oxidation. Many believe that taking antioxidant supplements can slow the aging process by preventing free radical damage. There are plenty of studies to back up this point of view. Every indication is that the typical diseases of aging can largely be prevented and avoided by leading a healthy lifestyle and taking antioxidants. For example, in a study from the Harvard School of Public Health, more than 130,000 healthy middle-aged and older adults who consumed at least 100 IU of vitamin E every day for two or more years had a reduced risk of cardiovascular disease.

As we age, our digestive systems become less efficient and we don't absorb nutrients as well. Taking vitamins, and particularly antioxidants, is an important key to preventing age-related diseases caused by nutritional deficiencies.

A Canadian study of 96 healthy people over age 65, found that those who took a multivitamin containing the RDA (Recommended Daily Allowance) of vitamins and minerals, plus slightly higher levels of vitamin E and beta-carotene, had stronger immune systems and half as many infections as those taking placebos. I hope that in the future we have RDAs for children, teenagers, adults and senior citizens, that will specifically address the needs of each age group.

ANTIOXIDANTS AND CARDIOVASCULAR DISEASE

Staying free of heart disease involves more than just taking care of your heart. You need to take care of your entire cardiovascular system, including your arteries, veins and capillaries, as well as the blood that runs through them.

Antioxidants go to work in all these areas of the body to prevent aging and disease. There are literally dozens of studies showing these protective effects. For example, the Scottish Heart Health Study, which is tracking over 10,000 middle-aged men, evaluated the intake of vitamin C, E and beta-carotene, and found there was a protective effect for all three antioxidants. High vitamin E levels proved to be specifically protective against angina.

In a smaller study that actually measured vitamin levels in 152 people ranging in age from 26 to 65, there was a significantly *lower* rate of coronary heart disease in those who had *higher* levels of vitamins A, C, E and beta-carotene.

One of the primary roles of antioxidants in the cardiovascular system is to protect LDL or "bad" cholesterol from oxidation. According to a report out of the University of Texas Southwestern Medical Center, animal and human studies have shown that antioxidant supplementation with vitamin E reduces the extent of LDL oxidation. Their work also underscores the importance of eating monounsaturated fatty acids such as olive and canola oil, and tropical oils such as coconut oil, rather than polyunsaturated fatty acids such as corn oil and other vegetable oils.

Other nutrients that reduce LDL oxidation include beta-carotene and vitamin C. A study published by the NIH (National Institutes of Health) set out to measure the power of antioxidants to reduce oxidation of LDL cholesterol. They evaluated 19 middle-aged people with high cholesterol (an average total cholesterol of 283 mg/dl and an LDL of 197 mg/dl), along with 14 control subjects of similar age and normal cholesterol. The high-cholesterol group received a daily dose of 30 mg of beta-carotene, 1000 mg of vitamin C, and 800 IU of vitamin E. After 1 month of the vitamin therapy, the onset of LDL oxidation was prolonged by 71 percent, and the rate of oxidation was decreased by 26 percent. This study showed that after 1 month of antioxidant supplementation, people with high cholesterol significantly reduced their susceptibility to LDL oxidation.

Many large epidemiologic (population) studies have been done comparing diet, cholesterol levels and rates of heart disease. There are populations groups in Europe that eat just as much if not more saturated fat than Americans, yet have less heart disease. Some of this difference may be due to their consumption of red wine, which is high in bioflavonoids, but there is increasing evidence that it is also due to their higher consumption of fresh fruits and vegetables.

ANTIOXIDANTS AND CANCER

Free radicals in tissues and cells damage essential body chemicals, and can harm DNA, the very building blocks of life. DNA damage can begin the process of cancer. Antioxidants are part of the body's natural cancer prevention mechanism, and supplements are a useful way to boost them. A major study in China showed that, over five years, a group that took 15 mg of beta-carotene, 30 mg of vitamin E and 50 mg of selenium per day showed a 21 percent lower risk of dying from stomach cancer.

Another study, comparing cancer-afflicted and cancer-free patients, showed that vitamin supplementation was associated with significantly reduced risk of basal cell cancer. In fact, the cost of supplementing the diet of the general population with antioxidants, like selenium and vitamin E, would be much less expensive and more appropriate than the treatment of the disease.

Several population studies have linked consumption of soy foods to a lower risk of certain cancers, including cancers of the breast, prostate, stomach, and lung. Soybeans, which I'll discuss as an antioxidant, contain many compounds generating great interest in the medical community including the isoflavones, some of which act as antioxidants.

ANTIOXIDANTS AND ARTHRITIS PAIN

Antioxidants have a profound influence on diseases of the connective tissue such as arthritis. Antioxidants can often play a large part in reducing the pain of arthritis, and can greatly cut down on the need for medications such as aspirin or acetaminophen which are used frequently to treat pain.

This was confirmed by a German study using the antioxidant selenium. The group using the selenium had far healthier joints than those who used a placebo. People with arthritis tend to be deficient in selenium.

The antioxidant vitamins E and C can also be deficient in connective tissue diseases, and both are extremely important in the development and maintenance of cartilage.

ANTIOXIDANTS AND EXERCISE

There's no doubt about it, exercise is definitely good for you. Less fat, increased bone density, and reduced heart disease and cancer risks are a few of its benefits. However, exercise does generate free radicals. This is a normal result of increased oxygen consumption and is not normally a problem, because the body's natural antioxidant systems are designed to handle the extra load. Unfortunately, the high level of pollutants in our environment and the nutritional deficiencies of modern diets mean that exercise can leave us with a minus balance in our antioxidant account.

The assessment of antioxidant status in exercising individuals and athletes can be important to maximizing performance and good health. Different studies show that over-exercise, heat and environmental pollutants can all increase oxidative stress. The key to keeping fit in today's world lies in backing up your body's own defense and repair systems before strenuous exercise.

It has been shown that taking 1,200 IU of vitamin E for two weeks before strenuous exercise creates a significant reduction in oxidation during the exercise. In male college students who have done exhaustive exercise, those who ingested 300 mg per day of vitamin E for four weeks had lower levels of chemicals suggestive of free radical damage immediately following exercise than those consuming a placebo.

The preventive role of antioxidants has also been

demonstrated in marathon runners. Those who take 600 mg of vitamin C per day for 21 days prior to a 42 km run have a lower incidence of post exercise respiratory tract infection.

Interestingly, one antioxidant important to serious exercisers, is at its highest levels in the organ crucial to any physical activity—the heart. This is the nutrient coenzyme Q10. Coenzyme Q10 works with vitamin C to protect LDL cholesterol in the heart from oxidation and helps prevent damage to the arteries of the heart. This is typical of the cooperative interaction of antioxidants.

If you're serious about exercise, I recommend that you also get serious about taking your antioxidant supplements!

THE "BIG THREE" ANTIOXIDANTS

In addition to the super antioxidants, I'll be telling you about what I call the "big three" stars of the vitamin antioxidant world: beta-carotene, vitamin E and vitamin C. They should be taken in addition to the super antioxidants, as they work hand in hand with each other. Every super antioxidant mentioned in this book works better with the "big three." Although I won't go into selenium in detail, it is a mineral antioxidant that should be included in your daily multivitamin, as it also works hand in hand with many of the other antioxidants.

Even mainstream medical doctors tend to agree these days that taking the "big three" will help you stay healthier. The "big three" stop or slow the oxidation process by neutralizing free radicals. These antioxidants also help the body fight disease and the effects of aging in other ways, yet Americans aren't getting enough of them. A study evaluating three national surveys of more than 13,000 Americans found that the majority of those surveyed were getting less than the RDA for these vitamins. (And the RDA is far less than I recommend!)

In a study at the University of Toronto, people with bladder cancer who took high daily doses of vitamins A (40,000 IU), B6 (100 mg), C (2000 mg), and E (400 IU), had 40 percent fewer tumors than a control group that took no vitamins, and also lived almost twice as long. Researchers concluded that high doses of vitamins may provide protection against the high recurrence rates that tend to be present with bladder cancer.

Doctors have used a combination of the "big three" antioxidants plus vitamin A and manganese, along with radiation and chemotherapy for small-cell lung cancer. Patients lived longer and tolerated chemotherapy and radiation better than the group not given antioxidant supplements.

The famous Harvard nurses' and doctors' study, which looked at the health of thousands of men and women over a period of many years, found that heart deaths were 60 percent lower in those who took vitamin E.

Another large, long-term study, called the Basel Study, found that when blood levels of vitamins C, E, A and beta-carotene were low, it affected the rate of death from cancer and heart disease. For example, people whose levels of vitamin C and beta-carotene were low were more likely to die of heart disease. What's more, vitamin E has been shown in several studies to be a definite help to those already suffering from heart disease.

It's easy to see that there is a wide range of diseases where supplements of the "big three" antioxidants have been shown to play a beneficial role. In some cases the doses needed haven't been very high. For example, a study published in the *Journal of the American College of Nutrition* showed that a moderate dose of just 300 mg of vitamin C daily reduced the risk of developing cataracts by 33 percent. Vitamin E in 400 IU daily doses also dropped the risk. That sounds like pretty good health insurance to me!

THE BIOFLAVONOIDS

Bioflavonoids are organic compounds found in plants that are turning out to be key to the power of super antioxidants. All of the super antioxidants I'm going to tell you about contain bioflavonoids as a major part of their active principles. These powerful substances reduce inflammation and pain, strengthen blood vessels, improve circulation, fight bacteria and viruses, improve liver function, lower cholesterol levels and improve vision. Vitamin C works much more effectively when combined with bioflavonoids.

Bioflavonoids are found in a wide variety of plants. Some of the best food sources are the white material underneath citrus fruit peels, peppers, and berries. Although bioflavonoids are not considered essential to life, and therefore are not classified as vitamins, it is becoming clear that they *are* essential to good health.

CHAPTER 2

Beta-Carotene:
The Colorful Antioxidant

Beta-carotene is a member of the carotenoid family of plant pigments and a powerful antioxidant. As well as helping to prevent heart disease and cancer, it prevents vitamin C from being oxidized or destroyed. Beta-carotene and vitamin C working in concert are especially important in protecting the eyes. Beta-carotene's protective effect is also seen in the mucous membranes of the mouth, nose, throat and lungs.

The carotenoids are the pigments that give vegetables such as carrots, squash, and tomatoes their bright colors. They also give flowers such as nasturtiums, pansies and sunflowers their yellow color. These compounds were first discovered in carrots, which is how they got their name. Scientists have found nearly 600 carotenoids. Of these, our bodies can use about 50 to create vitamin A.

A CARROT A DAY KEEPS THE DOCTOR AWAY: BUGS BUNNY WAS RIGHT!

Although I recommend you take a beta-carotene supplement daily, you can get 15,000 IU of beta-carotene by eating one carrot. By getting daily beta-carotene from foods you also get a full complement of carot-

16

enoids, not just beta-carotene. Studies have shown that lightly steaming carrots is the best way to maximize your absorption of the beta-carotene. I also recommend you eat a raw carrot every day. Make carrot sticks and have them for lunch, or grate the carrot into a salad. In the famous Harvard nurses study, eating one carrot a day reduced the incidence of stroke by 68 percent, and the rate of lung cancer by 50 percent! If a prescription medicine showed that kind of success it would be the best-selling drug in the world! Carrots also contain fiber, and lower cholesterol.

This is also a good reason to take a natural beta-carotene supplement, which comes packaged as part of the carotenoid family, rather than a synthetic one that just isolates the beta-carotene.

VITAMIN A AND BETA-CAROTENE

Vitamin A is occurs in two forms—preformed vitamin A, called retinol (found only in foods of animal origin), and provitamin A, better known as beta-carotene (provided by foods of both plant and animal origin). Beta-carotene is made up of two vitamin A molecules. When the body needs vitamin A it uses an enzyme to break the beta-carotene molecule in half, creating two vitamin A molecules. This is why beta-carotene is considered a safer way to get vitamin A, which can accumulate in the body and become toxic if taken in high doses over a long period of time.

BETA-CAROTENE AND HEART DISEASE

One source of evidence for the protective effect of beta-carotene comes from a study of doctors with heart disease. A subgroup of the Physicians' Health

Study of male physicians between 40 and 84 years of age, comprised 333 doctors with angina pectoris and coronary revascularization. Those assigned to 50 mg of beta-carotene on alternate days had a 44 percent reduction in all major coronary events, including death from heart failure. Those taking beta-carotene also had a 49 percent reduction in events connected with blood vessels, such as strokes, heart attacks, revascularization or cardiovascular death. The beneficial effect of beta-carotene appeared in the second year of follow-up in this study, showing how this antioxidant had prevented further fatty degeneration of the walls of arteries.

Data from a Netherlands study of 674 patients who had heart attacks supports the idea that beta-carotene plays a role in the protection of polyunsaturated fatty acids against oxidation. In this way, beta-carotene protects the heart muscle from further deterioration caused by the restricted blood flow which can result from this kind of oxidation.

BETA-CAROTENE AND CANCER

Dozens of published studies show that a high carotenoid intake is directly related to a decreased risk of cancer. A variety of population studies have shown that a *low* intake of carotenoids results in an increased risk of cancer. Carotenoids actually do even more than protect. This may be due to beta-carotene's unique ability to squelch free radicals, which can spur the process of malignant tumor formation.

In one study of 50 cancer patients, recurrence of cancer was prevented in a significant number of those who took beta-carotene and vitamin E supplements.

Beta-carotene and/or vitamin E have also stopped cancer in its tracks in a variety of studies. This was best demonstrated in clinical trials on oral cancer.

Over the past few decades, numerous studies have shown high levels of beta-carotene to be protective against many types of cancer, working not just to suppress cancerous cells, but also to completely prevent the onset of cancer.

People who are deficient in vitamin A/beta-carotene often have skin diseases that resemble precancerous conditions.

BETA-CAROTENE AND INFECTIOUS DISEASES

Vitamin A deficiencies are clearly related to a higher rate of infection and slower healing. There is a worldwide campaign on the part of health care workers to make sure that children in Third World countries are given vitamin A to prevent a long list of infectious diseases and deficiency diseases. Some estimates are that a few pennies' worth of vitamin A could prevent 35 percent of the deaths attributable to measles in Third World countries.

BETA-CAROTENE AND THE IMMUNE SYSTEM

One of the best ways to combat viruses is to boost the immune system and increase the number of T cells present. T cells play a critical role in attacking and eliminating viruses. A number of studies have shown that high doses of beta-carotene can raise T cell levels.

This makes it important in the treatment of those suffering from AIDS and cancer, as well as less deadly viruses such as shingles, herpes and the flu.

BETA-CAROTENE AND THE SKIN

Although too much beta-carotene will turn your skin an orange hue, too little will cause premature wrinkling and signs of aging. Various derivatives of vitamin A have been used to improve skin quality, but keeping your beta-carotene intake high will work even better as a preventive.

BETA-CAROTENE AND THE EYES

My mother told me to eat my carrots so I would have good eyesight, and there's plenty of truth to that advice. Deficiencies of vitamin A are associated with night blindness. There is also some evidence that high dietary levels of beta-carotene prevent cataracts.

WHAT IS THE BEST FORM OF BETA-CAROTENE TO TAKE?

I recommend you take a natural form of beta-carotene that most commonly comes from a sea algae called *Dunaliella salina*. It is usually referred to on vitamin bottles as *D. salina*, or as a "marine source" of beta-carotene. This form of beta-carotene is patented by the Henkel company, and may also be referred to by its commercial name, Betatene. Natural beta-carotene in supplements also comes from carrots and other food sources. When you take natural beta-carotene you get the whole family of carotenoids, rather than just the beta-carotene found in the synthetic versions.

ARE THERE ANY SIDE EFFECTS FROM TAKING BETA-CAROTENE?

If you take high doses of beta-carotene over a long period of time, your skin may turn yellow. This will not hurt you! However, I don't recommend taking it in a high enough dose to create yellow skin. As with everything, moderation is the key. Don't take beta-carotene if you're taking the prescription drug Accutane, a drug used to treat severe acne.

WHAT FOODS IS BETA-CAROTENE FOUND IN?

You know that carrots are a good source of beta-carotene, and you've probably guessed that any of the orange or yellow vegetables are good sources of this powerful antioxidant. Beta-carotene is plentiful, too, in yellow fruits such as apricots and oranges. Sweet potatoes, spinach and most green, leafy vegetables are also good sources. Green tea, too, contains beta-carotene.

HOW TO MAKE BETA-CAROTENE PART OF YOUR DAILY LIFE

I recommend you take 10,000 to 25,000 IU of beta-carotene daily, with meals. In fact, beta-carotene works best with fats, so if you take it at the same time you're eating fatty foods you'll get more benefit from it. You may get enough beta-carotene from a combination of eating fresh fruits and vegetables and taking a multivitamin. However, if there's any question of getting enough beta-carotene and the other antioxidants, please add an antioxidant supplement. This type of health insurance is no good unless you make the payments, and those payments are made in antioxidants.

How Beta-Carotene Could Help You

Prevent and reverse heart disease
Prevent and reverse cancer
Improve vision
Protect the mucous membranes of the upper respiratory tract
Lower cholesterol
Prevent cataracts
Improve immune system function
Shorten the duration of diseases
Prevent and cure skin diseases
Prevent age spots
Promote growth
Promote strong bones
Promote healthy gums
Help treat acne

CHAPTER 3

Vitamin C:
The Ultimate Preventive Antioxidant

Vitamin C (ascorbic acid) is one of the most important vitamins our bodies require and one of the most powerful antioxidants we know of. It also enhances the benefits of almost every other antioxidants. Since as *homo sapiens* our bodies don't have the ability to manufacture vitamin C, we must replace this precious vitamin every day of our lives in food or supplements, or suffer the consequences. Most animal life is able to synthesize its own vitamin C and manufactures between 1,000 and 3,000 mg a day. While beta-carotene works with the fats, vitamin C works with the watery parts of the body, including intracellular fluids, blood plasma, lung fluid and eye fluid.

Vitamin C makes vitamin E work better by recycling it. Scientists working with vitamin C in solution found it delayed by a factor of 10 the time taken to use up both vitamin E and beta-carotene from the start of oxidation.

One of the most extensively researched nutrients, vitamin C is also one of the most easily available. Naturally-occurring vitamin C always exists in association with members of another set of powerful antioxidants, the flavonoids, and they work best together.

VITAMIN C AND DISEASE PREVENTION

How many people do you know who consume the recommended five to nine vegetables and fruits per day? And if they don't, are they taking supplements? There is increasing support for the concept that higher amounts than the RDAs of vitamin C and other antioxidant vitamins are needed to fight infection and chronic disease.

An extensive review of the literature suggests that populations that consume higher than the RDA levels of vitamin C (which is 60 mg per day from foods and other supplements) have a reduced risk of cancer at several sites, as well as a reduced risk of cardiovascular disease and cataracts. Higher-than-RDA levels of vitamin C have been associated with normal cholesterol and blood pressure levels and reduced risk of cardiovascular death.

Research shows that increased consumption of fresh fruits and vegetables, excellent sources of vitamin C, even without supplements, leads to a dramatic reduction in the incidence of gastric cancer and hypertension leading to stroke. It is in this way, too, that vitamin C plays a major role in parts of Asia in lowering the risk of cancer of the esophagus. It is thought this is partly because vitamin C can neutralize and scavenge free radicals in the upper gastrointestinal tract.

Many controlled studies prove the value of vitamin C as a disease preventive. In addition, it's known to contribute to resistance against pollution in air, water and food and to support the manufacture of white blood cells and interferon. Even before it was isolated as a specific substance, the food sources of vitamin C received official recognition in the fight against disease.

You may know the story of "limeys." This was the nickname given to British sailors when, in 1753, the navy instructed all Admiralty ships to carry limes and fresh vegetables to prevent the debilitating disease called scurvy. Symptoms included livid spots on the skin, bleeding gums and exhaustion. Until the new orders, sailors' fare consisted mainly of bread and salted meat. The fresh rations had spectacular results. From 1,754 cases in just one naval hospital in 1760, there was only one in 1806.

Over 200 years later, much more is known about the beneficial effects of vitamin C, and the research continues. One study, reported in the *British Medical Journal*, covered 730 men and women with no history of cardiovascular disease and evaluated seven-day dietary records. In these elderly subjects the mortality from stroke was highest among those with the lowest vitamin C intake. This study followed up its elderly subjects over a 20-year period, revealing vitamin C status to be as strong a predictor of death from stroke as diastolic blood pressure. The study concluded what I always maintain, that a high intake of vitamin C should be encouraged in the elderly. But don't wait. Starting young brings the full preventive benefits.

Vitamin C and other nutrients could benefit the national economy, too. Many Americans have vitamin C intakes at levels associated with increased risks of degenerative diseases such as cancer, cataracts and cardiovascular disease. Today there is great concern worldwide, but particularly in the United States, about high and increasing costs of diagnosis and treatment of such diseases, not to mention the common cold and other infectious illnesses. Just applying what we know about micro nutrients like vitamin C would have a major impact in controlling and actually lowering the costs of medical care.

HOW LONG WILL VITAMIN C LAST ON MY SHELF?

Vitamin C is very stable in tablet form. Long-term and short-term tests indicate that, under normal storage conditions, commercial vitamin C tablets are stable for periods in excess of five years (95 percent potency retention). But I hope your vitamin C will never be around for this long!

VITAMIN C AND COLLAGEN

Vitamin C is essential for the formation of collagen in the body. Collagen is a protein substance which holds together the cells needed to make tissue.

Collagen is important to the body because:

1. It is necessary for structural soundness of bones, teeth, connective tissue, cartilage and capillary walls.

2. It plays a role in wound and burn healing. It is necessary for the formation of healthy connective tissue used by the body to knit together a wound or burn.

3. It may play an important role in protecting the body from infection. A current theory holds that healthy collagen means stronger tissue, which enables the body to resist invasion by disease micro-organisms.

VITAMIN C AND YOUR SKIN

After your skin is exposed to sunlight its vitamin C levels drop significantly. Cream or lotion with vitamin C in it can help you guard against skin cancer and wrinkles. Yes, you read it right, vitamin C on the skin will penetrate deeply into the skin, reducing the damage to your skin from ultraviolet light, and as a result, reducing the wrinkles formed when your skin is damaged. According to a study reported in the *British Journal of Dermatology*, vitamin C applied to the skin of pigs protected them from ultraviolet light damage. By applying the vitamin C to *your* skin you get 20 times more into your skin than if you took it by mouth (but do keep taking it by mouth!). Vitamin C applied this way penetrates into the skin and can't be rubbed, sweated or even washed off. The beneficial effects can last up to 20 days, but according to the pig study, the skin is most protected when the vitamin C is applied regularly.

VITAMIN C AND ALLERGIES

If I could only recommend one thing to help with allergy symptoms it would be vitamin C. Large doses of vitamin C can decrease allergic symptoms, especially a runny nose and cough.

It is the body's release of histamines that causes allergic symptoms such as red, itchy eyes and sinus congestion. Vitamin C performs an important antihistamine action in the body, making it a critical ally in fighting allergies. This essential vitamin, which many Americans are deficient in, works directly to lower histamine levels in the body and supports the immune system in many ways. If you suffer during allergy season, I recommend you take at least 1,000 mg of vitamin C three times daily, and if your symptoms continue or get worse, increase that to 1,000 mg every three or four hours.

VITAMIN C AND ASTHMA

Vitamin C, along with other antioxidants, has been shown to be beneficial for treating asthma and preventing attacks. Vitamin C is the major antioxidant present in the airway surface liquid of the lungs. It helps to open up the airways and liquefy the mucus buildup caused by the allergic reactions underlying asthma.

Many physicians have noted that vitamin C can diminish, if not prevent completely, the symptoms of byssinosis, a lung disease which strikes textile workers who breathe fiber dust. This was proven in an actual study in which textile workers were given 250 mg of vitamin C every few hours. Those who received vitamin C had significantly less incidence of the disease.

It's now known that low dietary intake of vitamin C puts people at risk from asthma. In fact, low levels of vitamin C are common in people with asthma. A report in the *American Journal of Clinical Nutrition* found that asthma sufferers unfortunately often show a decreased preference for foods containing vitamin C. The report also found that several studies have shown that vitamin C supplementation of one to two grams daily improves respiratory measurements in asthmatics.

Vitamin C crystals have been used to stop the development of an asthma attack, and in one study, athletes with asthma brought on by vigorous exercise had fewer asthma attacks when they took vitamin C just before and just after exercising.

There is evidence that exposure to oxidants produced both in the body and in external substances could be a causative factor for asthma, particularly in infancy.

VITAMIN C AND HEART DISEASE

Many, many studies have shown that vitamin C helps reduce cholesterol levels and helps prevent heart disease. Other studies have shown that those who have certain types of heart disease have lower levels of vitamin C in their blood. People who take vitamin C also show a much lower risk of life-threatening blood clots that can cause a stroke.

Myocardial infarction is a disease involving the death of heart muscle tissue caused by an obstruction of the blood supply. One study dealt with 500 patients with acute myocardial infarction were put on either a control or an intervention diet within 48 hours of the infarction. The intervention diet was designed to be antioxidant rich. Sure enough, vitamin C levels in the blood increased more in the intervention group than the control group. The intervention group had safer levels of harmful enzymes and, not surprisingly, lower levels of free radicals. This put the intervention group at less risk of death or further injury from their illness. It's clear that a diet rich in vitamin C and other antioxidants is a sensible precaution against heart disease.

VITAMIN C AND COLDS AND FLUS

Numerous studies have shown that vitamin C gives the immune system a big boost in its job of fighting off colds and flu. Other studies show that once a cold or flu is in progress, taking vitamin C can reduce the severity of the symptoms and shorten the duration of the cold. One study discovered that patients taking 1,000 mg of vitamin C (one gram) every day (and increasing that dose to 4 grams at the onset of a cold), had a nine percent reduction in the frequency of colds and a 14 percent reduction in sick days.

VITAMIN C AND CANCER

The protective effect of vitamin C against cancer is well established. Over and over again, in population studies, those whose diet includes significant amounts of vitamin C show a lower risk of most kinds of cancer. Other studies show that vitamin C actually blocks the formation of certain substances in the body that cause cancer. Small studies done on the ability of vitamin C to block cervical cancer show great promise, and more research is needed. Vitamin C has also been shown to reduce the ability of cancerous cells to form in the stomach.

Most of the research on vitamin C and cancer shows that vitamin C is a *preventive* more than a cure, but vitamin C can also assist if you're fighting cancer. Some researchers believe, as did the late Dr. Linus Pauling, that the studies on vitamin C and cancer already in progress have been flawed, and that better studies are needed.

VITAMIN C AND DIABETES

Diabetics who take vitamin C supplements can often reduce their insulin intake. One of the major complications of diabetes is the weakening of blood vessels, which can cause circulatory problems, infections and eye problems. Vitamin C has been shown to reduce these complications. Diabetics who are having kidney problems shouldn't be taking megadoses of vitamin C. If you have diabetes, please check with your doctor first before taking vitamins to reduce insulin intake.

WHAT'S THE BEST FORM OF VITAMIN C TO TAKE?

There are many forms of vitamin C on the market: buffered, esterified, with bioflavonoids, timed release, and ascorbates, to name the major ones. Vitamin C (ascorbate) as it is found in nature is combined with substances called bioflavonoids. Please take your vitamin C with ascorbate *and* bioflavonoids—they work best in combination.

Vitamin C is buffered, esterified or made in timed release form to prevent a common side effect of too much vitamin C, diarrhea. Timed release vitamins often cause gas or tend to pass right through the system without ever dissolving. The esterified forms of vitamin C work best to prevent diarrhea, but you can also buy the cheaper forms of vitamin C if you're willing to test your tolerance for it. You do this by increasing your dose of vitamin C until you get diarrhea, and then back off until it goes away. This will be the amount of vitamin C your body can use effectively.

HOW TO MAKE VITAMIN C PART OF YOUR DAILY LIFE

People are becoming more aware of the need to supplement their diets with extra vitamin C. Unfortunately, most people think that by taking an ordinary vitamin C tablet in the morning with their breakfast, they will be covered for the rest of the day. Actually, the vitamin C is metabolized and any excess is excreted in about two hours, depending on the quantity of food in the stomach.

It is very important to maintain a high level of vitamin C in the bloodstream, since it can be destroyed by stress, and any number of environmental pollutants, from cigarette smoke to carbon monoxide from exhaust fumes. You can do this by eating plenty of raw fresh fruits and vegetables (cooking destroys vitamin C), and by taking a vitamin C supplement with every meal. I actually recommend taking an antioxidant supplement that combines vitamins A, C, and E at every meal.

You should take as much vitamin C as your body can use without giving you diarrhea. When you are healthy, unstressed and in a relatively clean environment, your need for a vitamin C supplement will probably range from 500 to 3,000 mg daily. If you are ill, stressed or being exposed to pollutants and toxins, your need for vitamin C could increase by as much as 100 times the normal amount. As I explained above, try increasing the dose until you get diarrhea, and then back off from that a little until it goes away.

WHAT FOODS IS VITAMIN C FOUND IN?

Most fresh, raw vegetables and fruits contain at least some vitamin C. Cooking destroys vitamin C. One of the best sources of vitamin C is citrus fruit such as oranges and grapefruit. Kiwi fruit contains high levels of vitamin C. Other good natural sources of vitamin C are broccoli and red bell peppers.

How Vitamin C Could Help You

Prevent heart disease
Prevent cancer
Prevent stroke
Prevent allergies
Reduce inflammation
Diabetics may be able to reduce insulin intake
Protect against pollutants and other toxins

Shorten the duration of colds and flus
Prevent asthma and reduce severity of attacks
Protect the lungs from airborne pollutants
Protect the skin from sun damage
Reduce arthritis pain and inflammation

CHAPTER 4

Vitamin E:
The Healthy Heart Antioxidant

Vitamin E is one of our most important vitamins and a powerful antioxidant. If all Americans took vitamin E, it would save an estimated $8 billion a year in health care costs.

Vitamin E is another antioxidant, like beta-carotene, that works with the fats in our bodies. Vitamin E works most specifically to combat rancidity in our cells. Rancidity is caused when free radicals go after fat cells and oxidize them. Our cells contain membranes made of fatty substances called lipids, and vitamin E protects those membranes from free-radical damage. Vitamin E also works in our blood to neutralize free-radicals by absorbing their free electron.

The unsaturated vegetable oils are extremely susceptible to rancidity or oxidation, and eating them greatly increases our need for vitamin E to combat this oxidation. They literally start turning rancid as soon as the bottle is opened, and some of them may already be rancid. (In fact, as I noted earlier, I recommend that you only buy vegetable oils that are preserved with vitamin E, or add a capsule of vitamin E to your vegetable oil as soon as you open it.)

For over 25 years I have been urging you to take a supplement of vitamin E daily. Although scientists found vitamin E in the 1920s, and many nutritionists and scientists have also been recommending it for years, we are only recently scientifically proving beyond any doubt that vitamin E plays an important role in the maintenance of health, and particularly in a healthy heart.

VITAMIN E AND YOUR LUNGS

Vitamin E can help protect the lungs and other air passageways against environmental pollutants such as air pollution, pesticides, and industrial pollutants. In a recent study of nonsmokers, taking vitamin E was associated with a 45 percent lower risk of lung cancer.

VITAMIN E AND WOUND HEALING

Vitamin E is a powerful wound healer, and when it is used, scarring tends to be greatly reduced. Vitamin E has also been used successfully in treating burns. It accelerates the healing rate of burns and lessens the formation of scar tissue. When applied to the skin, the antioxidizing effect of vitamin E prevents bacteria from growing. The British medical journal *Lancet* reports that animal studies have shown vitamin E also helps lessen tissue damage. It's known, too, for its anti-inflammatory action and boosts the immune system's response to injury.

VITAMIN E AND HEART DISEASE

There are literally hundreds of good, solid scientific studies showing that vitamin E can prevent and even reverse many kinds of heart disease. Let's review just a handful of these studies.

A review of European populations cosponsored by

the World Health Organization (WHO) showed those with higher levels of vitamin E had a lower rate of coronary artery disease. The same result was true in the majority of countries in studies of European and non-European nations, even where saturated fat intakes were high.

Finland's Laplanders showed a 17 percent lower death rate from heart disease than their southern neighbors. A study of 350 people revealed a northern diet high in antioxidants, including vitamin E-rich reindeer meat!

The Nurses' Health Study of over 87,000 women showed that those who took vitamin E supplements greater than 100 IU per day had a 40 percent lower risk of coronary artery disease than those who took no vitamin E.

The Health Professionals' Follow-Up Study of over 39,000 males showed that those who took vitamin E supplements greater than or equal to 100 IU per day had a 37 percent reduced risk of coronary heart disease compared to those who took none.

A Harvard University study of 130,000 men and women found that daily doses of vitamin E of 100 IU or more taken for at least two years, resulted in a whopping 46 percent lower heart disease risk for women and a 25 percent lower risk for men.

Just 100 IU of vitamin E helped produce less constriction of heart blood vessels over two years in one group, compared to those not taking the vitamin. This was shown in a study at the University of Southern California School of Medicine. These results were supported by another study at the New Mexico School of Medicine of 440 patients who underwent successful angioplasty. During a three-year follow-up, patients who did not take vitamin E regularly saw almost double the recurrence of blood vessel constrictions of those who did.

The evidence grows for the beneficial effects of vitamin E to surgery patients. Another study from the University of California School of Medicine evaluated 156 men between 40 and 59 years of age who had a previous coronary bypass graft surgery. Results showed a reduction in coronary artery lesion for those taking vitamin E supplements.

A report in the *Medical Tribune* found that even at low doses, vitamin E came through as the heart's key protective nutrient. Even the medical establishment has jumped on the vitamin E bandwagon, with many MDs routinely prescribing it for themselves and their patients.

Here are a few of the effects vitamin E has on the cardiovascular system:

- Combats oxidation of cholesterol, preventing and reducing accumulation on the arteries.
- Is a natural anticoagulant, dissolving blood clots safely.
- Permeates the tiny capillaries, assisting in bringing nourishment to all body cells and thereby supplying oxygen to the muscles (especially the heart muscles).
- Prevents undesirable excessive scarring of the heart after an infarct, while it promotes a strong "patch" scar during the healing process.
- Is a natural vasodilator, meaning it opens up the blood vessels.
- Allows a greater flexibility in cells and muscles, preventing hardening of the arteries.
- Is an anticlotting agent that helps prevent blood clots in arteries and veins.
- Helps dissolve existing clots.
- Increases the blood's available oxygen (improves

the transportation of oxygen by the red blood cells).
- Reduces the need of the heart for oxygen by making the heart become a more efficient pump.

VITAMIN E AND DIABETES

Diabetics have been found to be able to reduce their insulin levels when given vitamin E. Some people with Type II diabetes have even been able to get off insulin completely by taking vitamin E supplements. (If you are diabetic, please check with your doctor first.) Since one of the main effects of vitamin E is its anticlotting effect, it can greatly aid in preventing the damage to blood vessels that frequently causes serious problems for diabetics.

Excessive levels of free radicals are a feature of diabetes and are possibly involved in triggering the disease. Three small trials reported by the American Diabetes Association all showed decreases in substances such as fatty acids in the blood vessels of diabetics given vitamin E supplements. Confirmation, again, of the important effects of this antioxidant.

VITAMIN E AND CATARACTS

It has been shown that a deficiency of vitamin E can contribute to the formation of cataracts and other vision problems. Supplementing your diet with vitamin E is good health insurance for the eyes. It works best when combined with vitamin C and selenium.

VITAMIN E AND CANCER

Vitamin E probably works best as a cancer preventive. The Chinese Linxian Study showed that 30 IU of vitamin E taken along with beta-carotene at 15 mg, and selenium at 50 mcg, lowers the risk of dying from cancer by 13 percent.

Vitamin E has been found to prevent the growth of breast tumors and can help protect against bowel cancer. In population studies, high levels of vitamin E in the diet have been linked to a decreased risk of lung cancer and stomach cancer. In one study, two groups of hamsters were exposed to a strong carcinogen. The group given vitamin E did not get cancer, and the group that did not get vitamin E all got cancer.

VITAMIN E AND NEUROLOGICAL DISEASE

One of the roles of Vitamin E has to do with proper neurological functioning of the body. Vitamin E has been found to be deficient in people who have many neurological diseases, including Parkinson's, cystic fibrosis, and epilepsy. There is some evidence that it may help alleviate or lessen the symptoms of these types of diseases in some people. Vitamin E is an oil- or fat-soluble vitamin, which means it can be stored in the liver. Toxicity studies have shown that 3,200 IU of vitamin E given daily to patients with Parkinson's disease did not have any side effects. This therapy did show a significant slowing of the progression of the condition. Some health practitioners believe that high doses of vitamin E can even prevent and reverse some neurological diseases.

VITAMIN E AND YOUR HORMONES

A vitamin E deficiency decreases the production of all pituitary hormones; of ACTH, essential to stimulate the adrenals, and the hormones which stimulate the thyroid and sex glands. With regard to fertility, vitamin E may help prevent free radical damage to the sperm.

WHAT'S THE BEST FORM OF VITAMIN E TO TAKE?

In nature, vitamin E is made of substances called tocopherols. Some vitamin E is made of just one type of tocopherol, such as d-alpha-tocopherol, and other kinds are made from mixed tocopherols. If you are over the age of 50, I recommend the d-alpha tocopherol in succinate (dry) form, because it is easier to absorb than the oil.

Vitamin E also comes as a oil, in its natural form. Whether the oil or dry form is best for you depends on how your body works. If you need vitamin E for problems such as dry skin, or hormonal balance, the oil form may work best.

There is a synthetic form of vitamin E called dl-alpha tocopheryl, which I *do not* recommend. It is not absorbed as well in the body and is also not as retained as well. In fact, I do not recommend any types of synthetic vitamins, as they put an unnecessary stress on the liver, which has to work harder to eliminate them.

HOW TO MAKE VITAMIN E PART OF YOUR DAILY LIFE

Vitamin E is not found in large amounts in any food, so it's a good idea to take a vitamin E supplement regardless of your diet. A *Lancet* report found vitamin

E to be very safe compared to other fat-soluble vitamins, with few side effects reported, even at doses as high as 3,200 mg daily. I recommend, though, that you take from 400 IU to 800 IU (dry form) daily, with meals and in combination with the other important antioxidant vitamins, C and beta-carotene.

WHAT FOODS IS VITAMIN E FOUND IN?

Vitamin E is found in dark green leafy vegetables such as broccoli and kale, as well as in soybeans, eggs, wheat germ, organ meats, many of the nuts, and unrefined vegetable oils. Most vitamin E is made from soybeans.

How Vitamin E Can Help You

Prevent and reverse heart disease
Reduce oxidation of cholesterol
Increase fertility
Prevent damage to sperm
Support the adrenal glands
Enhance production of steroid/sex hormones
Support the thyroid gland
Speed wound healing
Decrease the risk of cancer
Reduce insulin intake in diabetics
Prevent capillary damage in diabetics
Decrease scarring
Lessen the symptoms of some neurological diseases
Prevent cataracts
Prevent macular degeneration
Protect the lungs against airborne pollutants

CHAPTER 5

PCO'S:
The "Do Everything" Super Antioxidants

Now that you know something about how antioxidants work, I want to tell you about the "super" antioxidants; the most powerful free radical fighters known. The star of the super antioxidants is a complex of substances called proanthocyanidins, known for short as PCO's. I've told you how important bioflavonoids are to your health, and PCO's rank as our most powerful flavonoids.

If you suffer from memory loss, varicose veins, diabetes, heart disease, arthritis, high cholesterol, allergies, or macular degeneration, I recommend that you try taking a PCO supplement. I have received more rave reviews for this product from people with the above illnesses than anything else I've recommended in years.

PINE BARK TEA GOT INDIANS AND SAILORS THROUGH THE WINTER

For centuries, sailors exploring the world feared one thing more than typhoons and sea monsters, and that was scurvy, a fatal disease caused by vitamin C deficiency. In those days however, they had no idea that their diet of biscuits and salted meat was causing the

42

disease. Early scientists who suggested lack of fresh fruits and vegetables might be the problem were laughed at and called quacks.

When the French explorer Jacques Cartier became trapped in the ice on the St. Lawrence river in the winter of 1534, his 110-man crew began dying of scurvy. Some 25 of them had died of this horrible disease, and 40 were not far from death, covered with sores and suffering from weakness, rotting gums and swollen legs. A passing Indian named Agaya gave Cartier a tea made from pine bark, claiming it would cure the men of just about anything they were ailing from. Sure enough, the tea worked, and the men rapidly recovered.

A MODERN RESEARCHER DISCOVERS GRAPE SEED EXTRACT

Some four centuries after pine bark tea saved Cartier's men, Professor Jacques Masquelier of the University of Bordeaux, France, read Cartier's account of the expedition and decided to study the components of pine bark. His research led him to identify substances called pycnogenols, a generic term he used to describe a large group of what are now called proanthocyanidin complexes. He later found the proanthocyanidins were in grape seed, lemon tree bark, peanuts, cranberries and citrus peels. Groups of these molecules, now called oligomeric proanthocyanidin complexes (OPC's) or procyanidolic oligomer (PCO's), were found to be even more potent. (I call them PCO's.)

With all the wine-making in France, Masquelier soon found that grape seeds were a cheaper and more potent source of PCO's than pine bark. He and others carried out extensive research on PCO's using grape seed extract.

The term "pycnogenol" is now a registered commercial trademark of a Swiss company that sells PCO supplements extracted from pine bark. I personally recommend grape seed extract because most PCO research was done with grape seeds, it is more potent than pine bark, and it is less expensive.

THE MOST POTENT ANTIOXIDANT KNOWN

Extensive research done on the PCO extract from grape seed between 1951 and the late 1970s has shown it to be one of the most potent antioxidant substances known. It is 50 times more powerful at scavenging free radicals than vitamin E, and 20 times more powerful than vitamin C. Furthermore, it enhances the potency of both these vitamins.

PCO'S INCREASE VITAMIN C LEVELS

In addition to its ability to neutralize free radicals, grape seed extract strengthens capillaries, veins and arteries, increases intracellular vitamin C levels, and strengthens collagen, the basic building block of our skin, tendons, ligaments and cartilage.

PCO'S PREVENT HEART DISEASE

I predict that in the not-too-distant-future, we will be measuring antioxidant levels rather than cholesterol levels to predict the risk of heart disease. Nearly every symptom related to heart disease, such as a high level of oxidized LDL cholesterol, has a deficiency of antioxidants as its root cause. PCO's work specifically to stop "bad" cholesterol from forming, oxidizing, and sticking to your artery walls. They also work to prevent the artery damage that attracts oxidized cholesterol, and lower the overall level of LDL cholesterol.

A number of studies have shown red wine to be protective against heart disease. Researchers agree that it's most likely that the proanthocyanidins found in red wine that carry the protective factor. Another long-term heart disease study published in the prestigious medical journal *Lancet* showed that the higher the bioflavonoid intake, the lower the risk of heart disease, and conversely, the lower the bioflavonoid intake, the higher the risk of heart disease.

Only relatively recently have the benefits of PCO's for a healthy heart become known. Scientists exploring the antioxidant abilities of PCO's found that these substances work on many fronts to nip oxidation reactions in the bud. They have the basic antioxidant ability to neutralize free radicals by trapping them. But PCO's are unique in their ability to not only neutralize a wide variety of free radicals in different stages of activation, but to actually *prevent* free radical formation before it begins. PCO's can neutralize the free radicals associated with the byproducts of cellular energy production, with rancid fats and oils, with excess iron, and with tissue inflammation and degradation. All these types of oxidation reactions can contribute to heart disease.

Add this potent ability to wipe out all types of free radicals to PCOs' ability to strengthen blood vessels and capillaries in particular, and you have a powerful weapon against heart disease.

PCO'S IMPROVE CIRCULATION

The fact that PCO's strengthen blood vessels makes them very important in reducing your risk of ailments associated with weak blood vessels, such as certain types of stroke. All diabetics, who nearly always eventually suffer from diseases of poor circulation, should be taking some type of bioflavonoid daily. Since PCO's seem to have the best ability to strengthen blood vessels, they should be at the top of the list.

The rupture of small blood vessels in your legs, called varicose veins, can be unsightly and uncomfortable, but the rupture of veins in your brain can be debilitating or even deadly. If you are at risk for a stroke, or have had one, I highly recommend you make PCO's a permanent part of your daily supplement routine.

If you have varicose veins, PCO's could be your key to preventing any further formation. Of course I'd also like you to get some daily exercise, drink plenty of water and eat plenty of fiber (one major cause of varicose veins is straining to have a bowel movement).

PCO'S PROTECT AGAINST STROKE

Most strokes occur when the blood gets "sticky" and clots, creating a logjam effect in an artery to the brain or in the brain. PCO's help prevent "platelet aggregation," the process of clotting that can lead to a stroke.

PCO'S IMPROVE VISION

A primary reason that eyesight fails as we age is that the blood supply becomes reduced. This can happen because capillaries rupture or become weak and unable to supply the eye with oxygen and nutrients. Two of the most crippling of these types of eye disorders are diabetic retinopathy and macular degeneration. Both have responded to PCO's in studies with humans.

PCO's also improve other aspects of eye health. In one study, 100 volunteers with healthy eyes received 200 mg per day of PCO or a placebo for 5-6 weeks, and a control group received no treatment. The PCO group had significant improvement in their night vision and after-glare vision compared to the placebo group.

PCO'S MAXIMIZE ATHLETIC PERFORMANCE

PCO's are also very useful for athletes looking to maximize their performance and minimize tissue damage. While they are enhancing the ability of your blood to deliver oxygen to your cells by improving capillary action, they are also keeping your tissue strong and elastic and promoting rapid healing to tissues that may have been damaged by overexertion.

PCO'S KEEP YOU LOOKING AND FEELING YOUNG

Scientists who study the process of aging tend to agree that oxidation reactions are one of the primary causes of aging and diseases related to aging. Thus it only makes sense to protect against the physical toll the years take by taking antioxidants. In that regard, because they are so potent and their effects are so wide-ranging, PCO's may be one of our best antiaging supplements. They will work to keep your skin looking young, increase energy, and improve flexibility. They are protective against heart disease, cancer, stroke and arthritis, the major diseases of the elderly.

HOW TO TAKE PCO'S

If you're over the age of 50, I recommend you include 50 mg of PCO's in your daily supplement regimen as an antiaging and preventive measure. If you're using it therapeutically for a specific ailment, you can take 150-300 mg daily.

I recommend the grape seed PCO extract that comes in a "phytosome" package, meaning that the molecules are combined with phosphatidylcholine, a natural component of lecithin. This new process allows the body to absorb and utilize much more of the PCO than it would otherwise.

How PCO's Could Help You

Lower your risk of heart disease
Strengthens capillaries and blood vessels
Increases vitamin C levels
Inhibits the destruction of collagen (the substance that holds the skin together)
Strengthens tendons, ligaments and cartilage
Reduce inflammation caused by arthritis
Improve athletic performance by minimizing tissue injury and inflammation
Enhance immune response
Promote faster healing
Combat cancer
Retard the aging process
Greater flexibility
Lower your risk of heart disease

Promote healthy, beautiful skin
Reduce water retention and bloating
Increase resistance to bruising
Reduce susceptibility to colds and flus
Improve night vision
Improve "after glare" vision
Improve overall vision
Prevent cataracts and macular degeneration
Reduce PMS symptoms
Enhance energy
Improve memory
Improve resistance to radiation
Improve resistance to environmental toxins
Reduce or eliminate allergy symptoms

CHAPTER 6

Green Tea:
The Anticancer and Antivirus Super Antioxidant

Super antioxidants can come from unexpected sources. Whoever would guess that a humble little cup of green tea could protect you from cancer, heart disease, viruses and a long list of other ills? That's right, green tea, the most popular of Asian drinks, turns out to have a long list of health benefits. And by the way, being the most popular Asian drink also makes green tea the most widely consumed beverage on the planet after water—some 2.5 million tons a year!

HAVE A CUP OF ANTIOXIDANTS

A British study evaluating the antioxidant activity of green tea, pouchong tea, oolong tea and black tea extracts found that all of the tea extracts showed antioxidant activity.

The antioxidants specific to green tea are polyphenols, bioflavonoids that act as super antioxidants by neutralizing harmful fats and oils, lowering cholesterol and blood pressure, blocking cancer-triggering mechanisms, inhibiting bacteria and viruses, improving digestion, and protecting against ulcers and strokes. The specific type of polyphenol found in green tea is called a catechin.

50

About half of the polyphenols in green tea are epigallocatechin gallate (EGCG), the most biologically active polyphenol. Other ingredients in green tea include the amino acid theanine, carotenoids, chlorophyll and the proanthocyanidins also found in grape seed extract, pine bark, bilberry and ginkgo.

While there are 3,000 varieties of tea in the world, it is the variety called *Camellia sinensis* that is consumed in such quantities and has the health benefits. In the West we're familiar with Camellia sinensis as black teas such as Earl Grey, orange pekoe and English breakfast, which are crushed before drying to allow some fermentation to take place. Green tea comes from the same plants, but is simply picked and dried without fermentation, allowing more of the original catechin content to remain intact. Oolong is a semi-fermented tea that falls in between black and green tea. Green tea contains 30-42 percent catechins, Oolong tea contains 8-20 percent catechins, and black tea contains 3-10 percent catechins.

A cup of green tea contains about 35-50 mg of caffeine. In contrast, a cup of coffee contains 75-95 mg of caffeine. Contrary to popular opinion, tea does not contain tannins. It is the polyphenols that give it the acrid taste which reminds us of tannins.

GREEN TEA INHIBITS CANCER

The studies showing that green tea inhibits cancer are impressive. In one, the lung cancer rate in mice fed green tea was reduced by 45 percent. Other animals studies suggest that green tea can cut the rate of stomach and liver cancer and slow the progress of skin cancer.

In Shizuoka province in Japan, where green tea is produced and heavily consumed by residents, cancer rates are sharply lower than those in other parts of the country. Green tea's protective effect may also explain why lung cancer rates are lower among Japanese smokers than American smokers.

Because the rate of breast cancer is so low in Japan, much research has been done to find out whether green tea plays a protective role. Animal studies, population studies and anecdotal evidence all suggest that green tea contributes significantly to Japan's lower breast cancer rates. In the largest study comparing the power of a variety of antioxidants to block breast cancer in animals, green tea catechins were the most potent inhibitors of the cancer.

Green tea has also been tested for its ability to protect against skin cancer, and once again came out a winner.

You've probably heard that substances called HCA's (heterocyclic amines) formed during the cooking, and especially charring, of meat can be carcinogenic. Well, have a cup of green tea with your char-broiled meat, because green tea neutralizes those substances in the stomach. In one study, EGCG's (making up, as noted earlier, about half the catechin content of green tea) were 85 percent effective in reducing the formation of HCAs. Now, that's potent stuff!

With the wide variety of testing that has been done on green tea's cancer-blocking effects, I think it's safe to assume that green tea can make a significant positive difference with just about every type of cancer.

Researchers believe that green tea blocks the progression of cancer by blocking the formation of cancer-causing compounds, suppressing the activation of already-present carcinogens, and by trapping and neutralizing toxins that could promote cancer.

But green tea doesn't just stop the cancer from ever getting started, it can also stop tumor growth in its tracks. According to Japanese studies, very low doses of green tea added to the water of laboratory rats prevented colon cancer, and an extract of EGCG prevented liver tumors from forming. A Chinese study showed that green tea powerfully inhibited intestinal cancer in rats.

GREEN TEA KEEPS VIRUSES AT BAY

The Chinese have studied various green tea extracts against many viruses, among them a form of HIV, hepatitis and herpes viruses. In every case, the extracts significantly inhibited the activity of the viruses. This indicates that green tea enhances the ability of the immune system to stop viral attacks. Adding plenty of green tea to your winter diet should help keep the flu at bay.

GREEN TEA PROMOTES A HEALTHY HEART

Like other polyphenols, green tea adds to your healthy heart by preventing the oxidation of LDL cholesterol and raising the level of "good" HDL cholesterol. As a bonus it also lowers triglyceride levels. In fact, in a series of Japanese studies, green tea extracts prevented oxidation in fatty substances better than glutathione, vitamin C, synthetic vitamin E (dl-alpha tocopherol) and BHT, a synthetic antioxidant often used as a food preservative.

GREEN TEA PROTECTS THE BRAIN AND LIVER

It's important to keep your liver in tip-top shape so it can efficiently dispose of waste and toxins in the body, and green tea has been shown to be protective of the liver.

The same mechanism that protects your liver protects your brain from oxidized fatty acids. One study showed it to be 200 times more protective against oxidation in the brain than vitamin E.

GREEN TEA IS AN ANTIBACTERIAL

Maybe we should add green tea to our municipal drinking water instead of chlorine, because it powerfully protects against nearly all types of bacteria, including cholera, salmonella and typhoid. And unlike antibiotics, green tea is selective about what bacteria it kills, leaving the "good" intestinal bacteria such as acidophilus, and going after those that cause digestive disturbances and damage.

GREEN TEA CURES GUM DISEASE

A dentistry school in Japan tested the effectiveness of green tea in reducing gum disease, and found that in some people it completely cured severe gum disease.

HOW TO MAKE GREEN TEA PART OF YOUR DAILY LIFE

There are a variety of ways to integrate green tea into your daily diet. One is to have a cup or two of the hot brew in the morning. In fact, replacing coffee with green tea might be one of the healthiest moves you could make. And you can replace iced black tea with iced green tea.

If sipping beverages isn't your cup of tea (sorry), you can find green tea extract in capsules at your health food store.

You need to drink a lot of green tea—10-20 cups a day—to take complete advantage of green tea's protective properties. Since that's way too much for most people (and more caffeine than I would recommend), if you have a specific illness that you want to prevent or treat with green tea, I recommend using the extract.

Ten to twenty cups a day represents about 1-2 grams of polyphenols, 0.5-1 gram of EGCG, and 0.5-1 gram of caffeine. The extracts contain a higher concentration of polyphenols and a lower concentration of caffeine. I would recommend taking one to two tablets or capsules of 30 percent polyphenol green tea extract daily, with meals, for disease treatment and prevention.

How Green Tea Could Help You

Protect against breast cancer
Protect against lung cancer
Protect against colon cancer
Protect against liver cancer
Protect against intestinal cancer
Protect against skin cancer
Protect against stomach cancer
Prevent oxidation reactions in the brain
Antibacterial against harmful digestive bacteria
Cure gum disease
Lower oxidized LDL cholesterol
Raise HDL cholesterol
Lower triglycerides
Inhibit viruses, such as HIV, hepatitis and herpes
Antioxidant protection against damaged arteries

CHAPTER 7

Ginkgo Biloba:
The Better Memory and Circulation Super Antioxidant

Ginkgo biloba is an herb that comes from one of the most ancient species of trees on the planet. These magnificent trees, which can grow to be huge, have been around for at least 300 million years! Some people refer to it as a "living fossil." It's so old, that it has no known living relatives—ginkgo is an entity unto itself. The very properties that have helped ginkgo survive over the millennia may very well be the same properties that give it such potent medicinal value. Ginkgo is sacred to the Buddhists, and features prominently in Chinese and Japanese medicinal folklore.

You've probably seen ginkgo trees on the sidewalks of American city streets, where they are used both for their decorative value, and their ability to withstand the ravages of air pollution, periods of heavy drought or rain, and competition from concrete sidewalks. The leaves have a distinctive fan shape with parallel veins, and are divided up the middle.

The Chinese have been using ginkgo leaf medicinally for at least 5,000 years. They prize ginkgo leaves for their ability to improve blood flow to the brain, open up congested lungs, and improve blood flow to the extremities.

In the past decade or so, this amazing plant has been as well studied and researched as most pharmaceutical drugs. Ginkgo has been the subject of over

300 scientific studies. It is one of the best-selling medicines in Europe, sold to an estimated 10 million people there every year. GBE, a standardized ginkgo biloba extract, is a government-approved medicine in Germany and is covered by health insurance there. Ginkgo was given a major review article in the prestigious British medical journal *Lancet*, with the suggestion that it may be a powerful antiaging aid, particularly in regard to improving brain function.

WHAT MAKES GINKGO TICK

In general, ginkgo's healing abilities have to do with improving circulation and improving the flow of oxygen to the brain and extremities. However, its spectrum of activities is wide, thanks to the wide variety of substances it contains, including flavonoids, terpenoids (ginkgolides, bilobalide), ginkgo heterosides, proanthocyanidins (PCO's) and organic acids.

GBE, the standardized extract most widely used in Europe, contains 24 percent flavonoid glycosides and 6 percent terpenes.

The flavonoids scavenge free radicals, protect against cell membrane damage, and inactivated harmful enzyme reactions. Ginkgolides can protect against stroke by keeping certain parts of the blood from clumping or clotting, and bilobalide may inhibit swelling of the brain. You're familiar with the PCO's, which in combination with the other ingredients in ginkgo, reduce blood pressure.

GINKGO IMPROVES CIRCULATION, ESPECIALLY FOR DIABETICS

In addition to improving circulation to the extremities, ginkgo improves "microcirculation," which is the blood flow into the tiny capillaries feeding into larger blood vessels. This makes it useful for treating vision problems such as cataracts, macular degeneration, varicose veins, cold or numb feet and hands, and ringing of the ears (tinnitus).

One of my favorite ginkgo stories is of an elderly diabetic man who had a sore on his big toe that was down to the bone and wouldn't heal. His doctors wanted to amputate his foot. Naturally he had some resistance to that idea, so he decided to try some ginkgo as a last resort. Within ten days his toe had healed and his foot was a rosy pink color instead of its usual gray.

Ginkgo improves the symptoms of peripheral vascular disease, such as pains in the legs at night, cramps, numbness and impotence. Studies show that taking ginkgo for several weeks, up to six months, brought about a 48-68 percent increase in walking distance.

Ginkgo's ability to improve blood flow to the brain and strengthen blood vessels contributes to its ability to protect against strokes caused by weakened blood vessels.

GINKGO CAN HELP DIZZINESS, VERTIGO AND TINNITUS

The above symptoms tend to go together, and ginkgo has been found to be effective in treating all of them, as well as the symptoms that tend to accompany vertigo, such as nausea, vomiting, headaches and hearing difficulty. Those who suffered from vertigo were able to travel, turn their head and bend down without symptoms. The patients in the studies were given 60-160 mg of ginkgo extract daily, and consistently showed a 40-80 percent improvement after one to three months of treatment. Even cases caused by disease or injury tended to respond favorably to ginkgo. These symptoms can be caused by impaired blood flow to the inner ear, making ginkgo the perfect medicine.

GINKGO BOOSTS BRAIN POWER

Ginkgo's best-known and most noticeable effects are in improving blood flow to the brain, with the result of improving memory and cognitive (thinking) abilities. It is thought that a large part of this effect is created by the action of the terpenes present in ginkgo, particularly one called ginkgolide. Ginkgolide inhibits platelet-activating factor (PAF), which is known to weaken blood vessels, with the result of impairing blood flow to the brain.

Ginkgo is clearly effective and safe for treating what is called in medical circles "cerebral insufficiency," or impaired blood flow to the brain, particularly in parts of the brain where blood flow has been interrupted by damage. These effects also fall under the category of improving brain disorders caused by atherosclerosis, or blockage of blood vessels.

In some cases, ginkgo helps relieve and control the symptoms of Alzheimer's disease. This may be due to its unusual ability to enhance the effects of norepinephrine, which tends to be depleted in some areas of the brain in Alzheimer's patients.

In a French double-blind study of 166 patients with aging-related memory and cognitive problems, the treated group showed significant improvement compared to the untreated group after three months. The authors of the study noted that those who had the severest problems seemed to be those who were helped the most. The many similar studies done in

England and Germany produced similar results. Some of the aspects of brain function tested were orientation, communication, mental alertness, recent memory, and freedom from confusion.

Ginkgo can improve the ability to remember, the speed of memory and mental performance, as well as other symptoms of cerebral insufficiency such as headaches, dizziness, ringing in the ears, clumsiness and hearing impairment.

The benefits of ginkgo are not restricted to the elderly. Ginkgo extracts have become popular among college students writing papers and preparing for exams.

GINKGO PROTECTS AGAINST HEART DISEASE

Many of the same substances that give the other super antioxidants their heart-protecting power are found in ginkgo. In that respect, it lowers LDL cholesterol, reduces the amount of oxidized LDL cholesterol circulating, raises HDL cholesterol, and lowers triglyceride levels.

Ginkgo also protects against heart disease by improving circulation to the heart and improving the delivery of oxygen to the heart muscle.

GINKGO CAN CURE LEG CRAMPS

Intermittent claudication, a condition caused by restricted blood flow in the arms and legs, causes painful muscle cramping and difficulty walking. If you have intermittent claudication, keep walking as much as you can, because that will steadily improve your circulation. But you can also use ginkgo. In numerous studies, it has been shown to increase pain-free walking distance in those with intermittent claudication or any other circulation problems.

GINKGO PROTECTS THE EYES

Because ginkgo improves blood flow, it can also improve vision and prevent a range of vision problems caused by impaired blood flow, including cataracts. In both animal and human studies, ginkgo extracts decrease damage to retinal blood vessels induced by oxidation, and protected them from damage. The flavonoids present in ginkgo also contribute to its ability to strengthen the small blood vessels in the eye, improving both circulation and the delivery of other nutrients, including oxygen. When ginkgo was given to patients suffering from macular degeneration, 90 percent of the ginkgo group showed improvement in their vision, while only 20 percent of the control group showed improvement.

HOW TO MAKE GINKGO PART OF YOUR DAILY LIFE

Ginkgo may be one of our most important antiaging medicines. I know many, many people who swear by ginkgo and take it every day, and I recommend you do the same if you're over the age of 60.

Ginkgo biloba has a delayed onset of action and it may be a few weeks before you notice results, especially for problems such as tinnitus, which can take months to clear up. The effects of ginkgo do not generally show up after a single dose. It is not used in massive doses but in repeated doses that can produce beneficial effects over a relatively long period of time.

The best way to take ginkgo is in a liquid extract called GBE (ginkgo biloba extract) that is standardized. GBE is a concentrated and semi-purified extract designed to enhance ginkgo's health benefits and provide a consistent level of ginkgolides, the most active principles.

I recommend that you find a GBE extract containing at least 24 percent ginkgo flavoglycosides. You can take 60 tablets, 2-3 daily with food, or use the liquid preparations in a dosage of 1-3 droppersful up to 3 or 4 times a day, but check the label for recommendations.

How Ginkgo Biloba Could Help You

Improve memory
Improve balance
Improve ability to communicate
Improve dizziness
Improve headaches
Improve hearing
Relieve symptoms of senility
Prevent and cure leg cramps
Improve circulation
Strengthen blood vessels
Lower LDL cholesterol and oxidized LDL
    cholesterol
Raise HDL cholesterol
Lower triglycerides
Improve circulation to the heart
Improve circulation to the extremities
Prevent and improve effects of poor circulation in
    diabetics
Improve or cure tinnitus (ringing in the ears)
Warm up cold hands and feet

Improve vision
Prevent cataracts
Prevent macular degeneration
Protect against stroke
Protect against damage from head injuries

CHAPTER 8

Soy:
The Super Antioxidant, Anticancer Food

If I've already got you drinking green tea, perhaps you're ready to try something else from Asia! Many scientists believe that the frequent consumption of soy foods is a major factor in Japanese health and longevity. Soy contains a fascinating combination of beneficial chemicals, many of which have antioxidant properties that make this food one of nature's healthiest choices.

WHAT IS SOY?

Soy is the name for food made from soybeans. Soybeans are related to clover, peas, and alfalfa and are sometimes called soya. The beans are processed in different ways, making, for example, sauce, drinks and curds.

Soy is one of the few plant foods that contains the proper balance of the eight essential amino acids. This makes it a valuable protein source, especially since it is also low in fat and high in fiber.

THE ISOFLAVONE CALLED GENISTEIN IS SOY'S ANTIOXIDANT STAR

Isoflavones are compounds found in soy that contribute to its antioxidant powers. Study after study has shown just how effective isoflavones can be and one isoflavone in particular turns out to be a real star. Genistein came to the attention of the research community in the sixties. It has already been the subject of about 400 scientific papers, with more than 30 laboratory studies confirming that genistein inhibits the growth of cancer cells. The only source of genistein is soy.

One fascinating study found that when the diet of mice was supplemented with genistein for 30 days, there was a significant increase in the activity of antioxidants in their skin and small intestine. In another study Japanese researchers were looking for anticancer agents produced by bacteria. The most effective substance that resulted was not made by the bacteria at all—it was genistein and it was found in the soy medium used to grow the bacteria!

It's a fact that autopsies of Japanese men show that prostate cancer is as common in Japan as it is in the United States, but the cancer seems to grow much more slowly; so slowly in fact, that many men die without ever developing clinical disease. Now researchers suspect that genistein is blocking the growth of these tumors. A Finnish researcher and his colleagues compared the levels of isoflavones in Japanese and Finnish men. The levels of isoflavones were more than one hundred times higher among the Japanese men, with genistein occurring in the highest concentration of any other isoflavone. The researchers' conclusion, published in *Lancet*, was that maintaining a lifelong concentration of isoflavones in the blood could be the reason why Japanese prostate cancers remain latent.

A 1990 study by scientists at the University of Alabama showed genistein reduced the number of mammary tumors in breast cancer experiments on animals. The researchers found that genistein doesn't just block estrogen, but also cancer cell growth.

All these various studies and their results show that

genistein, unique to soy, its fellow isoflavones, and other important components of soy, are very interesting characters in the unfolding story of cancer prevention and protection.

SOY LOWERS CHOLESTEROL AND HELPS PREVENT HEART DISEASE

There have been hundreds of studies examining the effect of various forms of soy on blood fat levels in both animals and people. Most have shown that soy is a powerful cholesterol buster. Its antioxidants work to prevent LDL, or "bad cholesterol," oxidation and help reduce blood cholesterol levels.

In one ground-breaking study, laboratory rabbits were fed a cholesterol-free diet containing 38 percent milk protein. Despite the cholesterol-free regimen, the rabbits on milk protein eventually developed high cholesterol and severe thickening and hardening of the main heart artery. However, when the milk protein was replaced with soy flour, the cholesterol levels stayed low and the rabbits remained healthy.

A Japanese study published in the Annals of the New York Academy of Sciences found that the oxidation of LDL, or "bad," cholesterol was greatly reduced in rabbits fed on soy milk.

A study in Milan found a similar preventive effect in a group of volunteers who were all on low-fat diets and had high cholesterol levels. Those adding soy to their diets saw a drop in their cholesterol within just two weeks, while levels did not fall in those not eating soy. Even when cholesterol was deliberately added to their diet, soy eaters still experienced the same drop in cholesterol.

In rare cases children are born with a genetic tendency to develop extremely high cholesterol. In a recent study involving 11 children with very high cholesterol, researchers found that isolated soy protein could reduce LDL cholesterol more effectively than the standard low-fat diet. When isolated soy protein replaced the animal protein in their diet, the cholesterol levels dropped even further.

Soy is even given official recognition in Italy where the National Health Service provides soy protein free of charge to doctors for the treatment of high cholesterol. The evidence is in. Let's hope many more countries will choose to help soy play a similar role in heart disease prevention.

SOY CUTS CANCER RISK

There is significant evidence that diets containing large amounts of soy products are associated with an overall reduction in cancer deaths. There are good studies showing its preventive effect in cancers of the colon, breast, prostate, lung, esophagus and pancreas.

The proven anticancer effects of substances in soy are causing a real stir in the scientific community. Many studies have been prompted by the fact that Asian populations have markedly lower cancer rates than those in the West. Dietary factors are very important and are seen, for example in Asian immigrants to the United States who rapidly assume the risks of prostate cancer and breast cancer seen in Americans.

Possibly the most effective cancer blockers in soybeans are the isoflavones. They resemble the hormone estrogen, so they occupy estrogen receptors, but they don't behave like estrogens, which in excess are well-known carcinogens. Isoflavones are thousands of times weaker than the estrogens and actually act as anticancer compounds. This is similar to the way tamoxifen, the most widely used drug in breast cancer treatment, works. A study carried out in Cincinnati and England shows that isoflavones can be an effective treatment for premenopausal women with breast cancer and other cancers associated with estrogen.

A 1991 Singapore study, reported in *Lancet*, found that the risk of breast cancer in those who rarely ate soy foods was twice as high as for those who ate soy frequently. This was after all other food and lifestyle habits were accounted for.

A similar cancer comparison even shows up within the United States. A Harvard researcher found that Americans in South Dakota and Wyoming who regularly ate soybeans had less than half the risk of getting colon cancer as those who didn't eat soy.

The National Cancer Institute released a report showing that soy inhibits cancers of the mouth.

Some soy antioxidants are poorly absorbed in the intestines and go directly to the colon. Once there, these substances play an important role in reducing the development of colon tumors.

Japanese experiments with soy show that the antioxidants found in soy prevent cellular mutations which would lead to cancer. In the laboratory, soy antioxidants prevent cellular DNA from being attacked by carcinogens.

SOY REDUCES MENOPAUSE SYMPTOMS

Did you know there is no word to describe "hot flash" in Japanese? In fact many studies show that most Japanese women never experience a hot flash, and complain of far fewer unpleasant symptoms of menopause than do western women.

A recent Canadian study of Japanese women and menopause reported that hot flashes were mentioned by only 12 of the 105 women interviewed, and no one talked about night sweats. Another study compared menopausal Japanese, Canadian, and U.S. women. The Japanese women had far fewer physical and mental complaints than did the western women. While over 30 percent of both the Americans and Canadians experienced hot flashes, lack of energy and depression, the figures for the Japanese women did not go above 12.4 percent. In fact, researchers reported that few Japanese women were on hormone replacement, but they did use more herbs and herbal teas.

Many scientists now agree that diet, including the amount of soy products, is a major factor in accounting for results like these.

SOY LOWERS NEED FOR INSULIN IN DIABETICS

Diabetics can reduce the amount of insulin they need by including a product made from soybean fiber. It can also be useful in weight control. This was a discovery made by Dr. Yoram Kanter, head of the Diabetes Service and Research Unit at a hospital in Haifa, Israel.

SOY AND CATARACTS

A Columbia University animal study suggests that genistein has the ability to inhibit the formation of cataracts. This most probably reflects its ability to act as an antioxidant in the oxygen-rich parts of the eye.

SOY FOR HEALTHY KIDNEYS

People with kidney disease would do well to make soy their main source of protein. Soy is one of the few complete plant proteins, and has been shown to be much easier on the kidneys than protein derived from a meat diet.

SOY FIGHTS OSTEOPOROSIS

Osteoporosis is the thinning down of bones, leaving them weak and vulnerable to fracture. It is a disease of aging and is related to a variety of factors, including exercise, diet, protein intake and the production of hormones. Theoretically, Caucasian and Asian women, especially those who are thin-boned and petite, run a much greater risk of osteoporosis. However, even though Asian women are small-boned, they have far fewer hip injuries than do Caucasian women. In fact, Japanese women have roughly half the hip injuries of U.S. women, and women in Hong Kong and Singapore fare even better. Excess protein causes calcium to be leached from the bones. Soy consumption results in far less calcium loss than does animal protein. This was demonstrated in a study by the University of Texas Health Sciences Center. Volunteers replacing animal products with soy foods in their diet saw a 50 percent drop in calcium in their urine.

Other studies suggest that the isoflavones in soy may help retain bone mass. Recently, two University of North Carolina animal studies showed low-dose genistein was almost as effective as a synthetic estrogen in preventing bone loss in rats without a natural supply of estrogen.

HOW TO MAKE SOY PART OF YOUR DAILY LIFE

Japanese men consume between 40 and 70 mg of genistein per day. U.S. men eat less than 1 mg! We need to change those numbers for both men and women. I recommend you make soy part of your daily diet.

There are many, many ways to incorporate soy into your diet, from soy protein powders, to soy milk, miso soup and tofu. My book, *Earl Mindell's Soy Miracle* (Simon and Schuster, 1995), will give you lots of recipes and helpful tips on making soy a part of your diet.

Soy comes in many different forms including soy milk, tofu, tempeh, miso, soy sauce and flour. These are all made in different ways, including fermenting, soaking, and grinding, frying, steaming and sprouting.

Studies on which forms of soy confer the most health benefits show that tempeh and tofu are among the best ways to eat soy. Soy sauce contains the least amount of beneficial nutrients and is high in sodium, so I don't recommend you use it in large quantities.

Remember, soy can't do the job on its own. Make it a part of a diet low in fat, high in fiber and rich in other whole foods, and vitamins.

How Soy Could Help You

Prevent heart disease
Lower LDL cholesterol
Reduce menopause symptoms
Prevent many types of cancer
Prevent cataracts
Maintain healthy kidneys
Reduce diabetics' need for insulin
Help prevent osteoporosis

CHAPTER 9

Glutathione and L-Cysteine:
The Antiaging and Healthy Eyes Antioxidants

I call glutathione (known as GSH) the "triple threat" amino acid because it is a tripeptide made from the amino acids cysteine, glycine and glutamic acid, and because it defends the body against oxidation and toxins on three major fronts. This humble little protein is found in the cells of nearly all living organisms on earth, and its primary job is waste disposal.

GSH has three main detox jobs in the body:

1) When there are free radicals lurking about, threatening to start an oxidation reaction, GSH catches them, neutralizes them, passes them on (often to another antioxidant such as vitamin E), and begins the cycle anew;

2) In the liver, GSH latches on to toxic substances and binds to them, so the liver can excrete them without being damaged; and

3) GSH prevents red blood cells from being damaged by neutralizing unstable forms of oxygen.

We literally cannot survive without this miraculous antioxidant. GSH also plays a role in fighting cancer, stabilizing blood sugar, and cellular repair after a stroke.

As glutathione does its detox work, it transforms itself into a number of different substances, including an enzyme, while always retaining its basic structure.

Each substance has a different name, such as glutathione peroxidase and glutathione disulfide, but for the purposes of this chapter we'll use GSH or glutathione as a generic term for the whole spectrum of glutathione transformations.

GLUTATHIONE WORKS HARD EVERYWHERE IN THE BODY

Glutathione's antioxidant work is the front-line defense for preventing oxidation of LDL cholesterol, which damages the arteries. It's also crucial in protecting the lymphatic system and the digestive system from an overload of unstable fatty molecules. It maintains the integrity of red blood cells, and prevents damage to them. If glutathione levels drop anywhere in the body, the burden of toxic stress goes up.

Cells with decreased levels of glutathione are more susceptible to the harmful effects of radiation, free radicals and many pharmaceutical drugs.

In addition to the many benefits of glutathione listed below, supplementing it may be useful in modulating blood sugar in diabetics and in boosting performance in athletes. There is also evidence that raising glutathione levels in stroke victims can significantly reduce injury to the brain.

GSH is one of the most abundant substances in the body, and as long as we have a good supply of its building block cysteine (glycine and glutamic acid are rarely in short supply) and its cofactor selenium, it will be hard at work doing its detoxifying chores.

HOW WE DEPLETE GLUTATHIONE

GSH levels drop as we age, and can also be depleted by:

- Chronic diseases such as cancer and arthritis.
- An overload of rancid oils (such as polyunsaturated and partially hydrogenated vegetable oils).
- Overexposure to poisons such as pesticides.
- Pharmaceutical drugs that stress the liver such as acetaminophen (Tylenol) and aspirin.
- Since glutathione often passes off its neutralized waste products to antioxidants such as vitamin C and vitamin E, and needs the minerals selenium, copper and zinc to do its cleanup work, a deficiency of these vitamins can impair its function.
- Birth control pills and hormone replacement therapy.

USE CYSTEINE TO RAISE GLUTATHIONE LEVELS

Because glutathione is so unstable by nature, it is difficult to stabilize in a supplement. However, cysteine, when taken as a supplement, will raise glutathione levels. Cysteine is used routinely in hospital emergency rooms to prevent liver damage when people overdose on drugs or alcohol; to detoxify in cases of heavy metal poisoning, and to protect against the harmful side effects of chemotherapy and radiation. Cysteine is currently being used successfully to raise T-cell levels in AIDS patients.

The most commonly used form of cysteine is N-acetyl cysteine, known as NAC. It has been used in Europe for 30 years to treat a variety of lung diseases involving excess mucus production.

It is important not to take too much cysteine, since the body works hard to keep it in just the right balance.

Supplementation with selenium and vitamin E can also raise glutathione levels in the body.

GLUTATHIONE KEEPS THE ELDERLY HEALTHY

Glutathione levels drop as we age, which no doubt contributes greatly to the aging process and diseases of aging. A study done in England in a community of elderly people showed that low glutathione levels were associated with a 24 percent higher rate of illness and death, higher cholesterol, and higher body weight. Those who had heart disease, cancer, arthritis and diabetes had significantly lower levels of glutathione than those who were healthy.

Many elderly people suffer from malnutrition because they are unable to shop or cook healthy foods, or because their digestive system is working inefficiently and they aren't absorbing nutrients. This leads to a depletion of antioxidants in the tissues, setting the stage for cancer to take hold.

CYSTEINE BREAKS UP MUCUS IN THE LUNGS

NAC is used in Europe for coughs, asthma prevention and chronic bronchitis, because it is very effective at breaking up mucus in the lungs. A lung infection gets serious when the mucus gets so thick you can't cough it up. It is currently undergoing clinical trials in Europe to find out how well it works at preventing lung disease.

Cysteine liquefies the mucus, making it easy to cough up. If you have a tendency to get a winter cough, put some NAC in the medicine cabinet and take it at the first sign of lung troubles.

GLUTATHIONE/CYSTEINE BOOST THE IMMUNE SYSTEM

An important study done in Germany showed that HIV-infected humans and SIV-infected monkeys had low levels of cysteine and glutathione. Raising the levels of these substances increased T cells, a key marker of good immune system function. In the published study, the authors hypothesized that part of the mechanism that switches those who are HIV-positive into AIDS is very low cysteine and glutathione levels. I have heard a number of anecdotal reports that cysteine supplements are helping dramatically in HIV-infected people.

I would recommend trying cysteine supplements if you have any type of acute viral infection such as the flu, or a chronic viral infection such as herpes. While this is still experimental, there is enough clear evidence to warrant trying it.

If you're fighting a serious virus, please don't make the mistake of thinking that megadoses of cysteine will work better than recommended doses—you will only stress your body's systems further if you take too much cysteine.

GLUTATHIONE/CYSTEINE KEEP CANCER AT BAY

Some cancer researchers theorize that one way cancer gets a foothold in the body is by taking advantage of cell weakness caused by oxidation. When free radicals are running amok, it gives cancer cells an opportunity to get into a cell, damage its DNA, and get their own growth pattern going.

Some of ways glutathione and cysteine may prevent and reverse cancer are:

- Neutralize free radicals.
- Block the action of toxins that are carcinogenic.
- Prevent carcinogens from interfering with DNA.
- Prevent carcinogens from altering chromosomes.
- Suppress the action of cancer promoters such as excess estrogen.
- Suppress the growth of tumors.

A study done in India with women suffering from cervical cancer found the farther the disease progressed, the lower the levels of cysteine and glutathione dropped, and the higher the levels of lipid peroxides, harmful oxidized fatty substances.

A report from scientists in the Netherlands on using cysteine to treat lung cancer points out that tumor growth can only happen when detoxification pathways are saturated. They state that cysteine provides protection against mutagens and carcinogens at many different stages.

GLUTATHIONE/CYSTEINE PROTECTS THE DIGESTIVE SYSTEM

Glutathione also works hard to keep the digestive system healthy, neutralizing free radicals, particularly those caused by unstable fats and oils. It indirectly keeps the digestion healthy by being a key part of the liver's ability to detoxify the body. In a small Italian study of people with Crohn's disease, a serious chronic bowel disorder, it was found that levels of glutathione were much lower in those with Crohn's disease than in controls. Some preliminary data suggest that cysteine supplements may be useful in treating Crohn's disease and other bowel disorders.

GLUTATHIONE/CYSTEINE IS CRUCIAL FOR EYE HEALTH

The health of the eye, and in particular the macula, is dependent on a long list of antioxidants and their co-factors. This includes vitamins C and E and beta-carotene; the minerals zinc, selenium and copper; superoxide dismutase; glutathione and riboflavin.

We've known since the early 1900s that *all* people with cataracts have low levels of glutathione in the lens of the eye. In a study from the National Cataract Study Group it was reported that there was approximately a 35 percent reduction in cataract formation in the study group with the higher antioxidant levels. Another group reports a reduction in vision loss among those taking zinc supplements.

Low glutathione levels are also directly related to macular degeneration. The macula of the eye is an oxygen-rich environment where there's a large turnover of oxygen, generating a large amount of free radicals. Several studies have indicated that higher blood concentrations of antioxidants such as glutathione, beta-carotene, vitamin C and E are associated with lower levels of macular degeneration.

GLUTATHIONE/CYSTEINE PROMOTES HEART HEALTH

Underlying many of the risk factors for heart disease is a deficiency of antioxidants, which allows arteries to be damaged and oxidized cholesterol to float around in the bloodstream where it will attach itself to the damaged arteries. Glutathione is the body's first line of defense against oxidation of cholesterol. An Italian animal study even suggests that giving cysteine supplements after a heart attack could greatly reduce damage done to the heart.

HOW TO MAKE GLUTATHIONE/ CYSTEINE PART OF YOUR DAILY LIFE

Measuring glutathione levels is expensive at this time, but if you have heart disease, are at a high risk for it, or have high LDL cholesterol levels, I recommend you try raising your glutathione levels. The best way to raise glutathione levels is by taking a cysteine supplement, preferably in the more stable form of NAC (N-acetyl cysteine).

To convert the cysteine to glutathione, you also need vitamins C and E, beta-carotene, and selenium. One of the best food sources of cysteine is eggs, which I encourage you to eat a few times a week, since they are full of nutrition and in most people, won't raise LDL cholesterol, in spite of rumors to the contrary.

Other foods that contain high levels of cysteine include watermelon, onions, garlic, yogurt, wheat germ and red meat. The cruciferous vegetables such as broccoli, cauliflower and cabbage stimulate the body's production of glutathione.

The recommended dosage of NAC is 500 mg, 1-4 times daily. Over than amount can upset the balance of your body's chemistry just as much as a deficiency can.

How Glutathione/Cysteine Could Help You

Prevent cataracts
Prevent macular degeneration
Prevent cancer
Supress tumor growth
Detoxify the liver, cells and lymphatic system
Break up mucus in the lungs
Prevent heart disease
Prevent arthritis
Prevent diabetes
Stabilize blood sugar
Protect the digestive system
Boost the immune system
Slow the aging process
Boost athletic performance
Reduce injury to the brain caused by stroke
Reduce damage to heart from a heart attack
Reduce cholesterol
Protect red blood cells from damage
Prevent LDL cholesterol from being oxidized
Protect cells from oxidation damage

REFERENCES

Aebi S and Lauterburg BH, "Divergent effects of intravenous GSH and cysteine on renal and hepatic GSH," Am J Physiol, Aug 1992, 263 pR348-52.

Aw TY et al; "Absorption and lymphatic transport of peroxidized lipids by rat small intestine in vivo: role of mucosal GSH," Am J Physiol Jan 1992, 262 pG99–106

Aw TY et al; "Intestinal absorption and lymphatic transport of peroxidized lipids in rats: effect of exogenous GSH," Am J Physiol, Nov 1992, 263.

Balasubramaniyan N, et al, "Status of Antioxidant Systems in Human Carcinoma of Uterine Cervix," Cancer Letters, 1994;87;187–192.

Ceconi C et al; "The role of glutathione status in the protection against ischaemic and reperfusion damage: effects of N-acetyl cysteine," J Mol Cell Cardiol, Jan 1988, 20(1)p5–13

Droge W et al, "Functions of Glutathione and Glutathione Disulfide in Immunology and Immunopathology," FASEB Journal, 1994;8:1131–1138.

Enwonwu CO and Meeks VI, "Bionutrition and Oral Cancer in Humans," Critical Reviews in Oral Biology and Medicine, 1995;6(1):5–17

Flagg EW et al; "Plasm total glutathione in humans and its association with demographic and health-related factors," Br J Nutr, Nov 1993, 70(3)p797–808.

Fletcher RH and Fletcher, SW, "Glutathione and Ageing: Ideas and Evidence," The Lancet, November 19, 1994;344:1379–1380.

Iantomasi T et al, "Glutathione Metabolism in Crohn's Disease," Biochemical Medicine and Metabolic Biology, 1994;53:87–91.

Jendryczko A et al, "Effects of two low-dose oral contraceptives on erythrocyte superoxide dismutase, catalase and glutathione peroxidase activities," Zentralbl Gynakol 1993, 115(11) p469–72

Julius M, "Glutathione and Morbidity in a Community-Based Sample of Elderly," Journal of Clinical Epidemiology, 1994; 47(9):1021–1026.

Kinscherf R et al; "Effect of glutathione depletion and oral N-acetyl-cysteine treatment on CD4+ and CD8+ cells," FASEB J, Apr 1 1994, 8(6)p448–51.

Lassen KO and Horder M, "Selenium Status and the Effect of Organic and Inorganic Selenium Supplementation in a Group of Elderly People in Denmark," Scandinavian Journal of Clinical Laboratory Investigation, 1994;54:585–590.

Loguercio C et al, "Effect of S-adenosyl-L-methionine Administration on Red Blood Cell Cysteine and Glutathione Levels in Alcoholic Patients With and Without Liver Disease," Alcohol and Alcoholism, 1994;29(5):597–604.

Miura K et al, "Cystine uptake and glutathione level in endothelial cells exposed to oxidative stress," Am J Physiol, Jan 1992, 262.

Miura K et al, "Depletion of brain glutathione by buthionine sulfoximine enhances cerebral ischemic injury in rats," AM J Physiol, Feb 1992, 262.

Newsome, DA, "Role of Antioxidants in Macular Degeneration: An Update," Ophthalmic Practice, 1994;12:4:169–171.

Paolisso G et al; "Plasma GSH/GSSG affects glucose homeostasis in healthy subjects and non-insulin-dependent diabetics," Am J Physiol, Sep 1992, 262.

Pejaver R et al, "High-Dose Vitamine E Therapy in Glutathione Synthetase Dificiency," Journal of Inher. Metab. Dis., 1994;17:1749–1750.

Sastre J et al; "Exhaustive physical exercise causes oxidation of glutathione status in blood: prevention by antioxidant administration," Am J Physiol, Nov 1992, 263 (5 Pt 2) pR992–5.

Van Zandwijk NC, "N-Acetylcysteine for Lung Cancer Prevention," May 1995;107(5):1437–1441.

INDEX

Dr. Earl Mindell's

What You Should Know About . . .
series
in print or forthcoming

Beautiful Skin, Hair and Nails
Better Nutrition for Athletes
Fiber and Digestion
Health Benefits of Phytochemicals
Herbs for Your Health
Homeopathic Remedies
How to Create Your Personal Vitamin Plan
Nutrition and Stress
Super Antioxidant Miracle
Trace Minerals
22 Ways to a Healthier Heart